Carl Hanish

My Personal Emergency File
(If something is wrong with me ...)

In a nutshell the most necessary information for my family and friends

My Personal Emergency File (If something is wrong with me …)

Content

1 Disclaimer

Most of the suggestions in this booklet are based on common sense. Nevertheless, neither author nor publisher can accept any liability whatsoever. We ask for your understanding. In particular, references to legal matters do not constitute legal or tax advice.

For the sake of simplicity, persons and job titles are mostly used in the male grammatical form. Of course, all sexes are always meant. Discrimination against a gender is not intended.

And now I wish you perseverance when creating your emergency folder.

2 How to use this booklet

> **For each person a separate file has to be created. This is necessary to distinguish all facts and it helps with the inheritance tax declaration.**
>
> **In addition your family / friends should of course know that there is an emergency file and where to find it.**

Preparation:

1. Buy a new A4 folder per person.
2. Buy approx. 20 slip sheets and place them in each folder.
3. Label the back of the A4 folder with:
   "EMERGENCY FOLDER of first name last name"
4. Copy the pages from this book as many times as you need them and put them into the folder, with sections separated by slip sheets.

Content:

1. The content does not have to be beautiful, but it has to be readable, clear and informative.
2. You do not need a PC for this. When hand-writing entries, remember that someone has to be able to read the entries at some point.
3. As far as documents are to be filed, you can either file originals or copies, at will.

4. If there are separate folders for individual topics (e.g. insurance contracts), it is advised to indicate their location.

This template is not exhaustive. If something does not apply to you, just leave the space empty or cross out and enter something more suitable.

3 Personal Data

3.1 My Person

Surname	
First Name(s)	
Street, House Number	
ZIP Code, City	
Telephone 1	
Telephone 2	
E-Mail	
Date of Birth	
Place of Birth	
Gender	
Nationality	
Religion	
Marital Status	

Employer:

Company Name	
Contact Person	
Street, House Number	
ZIP-Code, City	
Telephone	
E-Mail	

3.2 My Spouse or Partner

Surname	
First Name(s)	
Street, House Number	
ZIP Code, City	
Telephone	
E-Mail	
Wedding Date	
Date of Divorce	
Matrimonial property regime, Marriage Contract	
Place of storage of the Marriage Contract	
Place of storage of the death certificate	

Surname	
First Name(s)	
Street, House Number	
ZIP Code, City	
Telephone	
E-Mail	
Wedding Date	
Date of Divorce	
Matrimonial property regime, Marriage Contract	
Place of storage of the Marriage Contract	
Place of storage of the death certificate	

3.3 My Parents

Surname	
First Name(s)	
Street, House Number	
ZIP Code, City	
Telephone	
E-Mail	

Surname	
First Name(s)	
Street, House Number	
ZIP Code, City	
Telephone	
E-Mail	

3.4 My Siblings

Surname	
First Name(s)	
Street, House Number	
ZIP Code, City	
Telephone	
E-Mail	

Surname	
First Name(s)	
Street, House Number	
ZIP Code, City	
Telephone	
E-Mail	

Surname	
First Name(s)	
Street, House Number	
ZIP Code, City	
Telephone	
E-Mail	

Surname	
First Name(s)	
Street, House Number	
ZIP Code, City	
Telephone	
E-Mail	

3.5 My Children

Surname	
First Name(s)	
Street, House Number	
ZIP Code, City	
Telephone	
E-Mail	

Surname	
First Name(s)	
Street, House Number	
ZIP Code, City	
Telephone	
E-Mail	

Surname	
First Name(s)	
Street, House Number	
ZIP Code, City	
Telephone	
E-Mail	

Surname	
First Name(s)	
Street, House Number	
ZIP Code, City	
Telephone	
E-Mail	

3.6 My Grandchildren

Surname	
First Name(s)	
Street, House Number	
ZIP Code, City	
Telephone	
E-Mail	

Surname	
First Name(s)	
Street, House Number	
ZIP Code, City	
Telephone	
E-Mail	

Surname	
First Name(s)	
Street, House Number	
ZIP Code, City	
Telephone	
E-Mail	

Surname	
First Name(s)	
Street, House Number	
ZIP Code, City	
Telephone	
E-Mail	

4 Persons to be notified

Who should be notified?	In Case of			
First name, Surname, Street, House number, ZIP Code, City, etc. Telephone, E-Mail	Accident	Hospital stay	Death	

5   Addresses of Friends

How does the person relate to you	First name, Surname, Street, House number, ZIP Code, City, etc.	Telephone number, E-Mail-Address

6   Addresses of Doctors and Consultants

How does the person relate to you?	First name, Surname, Street, House number, ZIP Code, City, etc.	Telephone numbers, E-Mail-Address
Notary		
Tax Advisor		
Laywer		
Family Doctor		
Caregiver/ Nursing		
Priest		

7   Health Insurance / Care Insurance

This information is important, so that the heirs can make pending bills.

Name of Health Insurance	
Contract number	
Contact person	
Street, House number	
ZIP Code,City	
Telephone	
Place of contract details	

Name of additional Health Insurance	
Contract number	
Contact person	
Street, House number	
ZIP Code, City	
Telephone	
Place of contract details	

Name of Care Insurance	
Contract number	
Contact person	
Street, House number	
ZIP Code, City	
Telephone	
Place of contract details	

Name of additional Care In-surance	
Contract number	
Contact person	
Street, House number	
ZIP Code, City	
Telephone	
Place of contract details	

8   Certificates / Documents / Numbers

In this section please attach copies of

- ID Card,
- Passport,
- Birth Certificate
- Baptism Certificate
- Marriage Certificate
- Divorce Certificate
- Death Certificate of the Spouse or Partner
- Leaving the Church Certificate
- Marriage Contract.

In addition, please enter here:

Tax Identification Number	
Social Security Number	
Church Membership	

9 Banks

In many countries Banks must report the assets existing on the day of death to the tax authorities.

Eventually your heirs can not access your accounts immediately. It is therefore advised to contact the bank on the subject of "proxy beyond death".

Name, Address and Telephone number of Bank	All Account Holders	IBAN / BIC	Type of Service
	Proxy granted to:		☐ Account
			☐ Deposit Account
			☐ Credit Cards
			☐ Asset Management
			☐ Loans
			☐ Bank Safe
			☐ Online Banking
			☐

Name, Address and Telephone number of Bank	All Account Holders	IBAN / BIC	Type of Service
	Proxy granted to:		☐ Account
			☐ Deposit Account
			☐ Credit Cards
			☐ Asset Management
			☐ Loans
			☐ Bank Safe
			☐ Online Banking
			☐

10 Pensions

Please list here all insurances / companies from which you receive a pension and tick the type of pension.

Name, Address, Telephone of Insurance or Company, Contract Number.	Statutory Pension	Widow Pension	Company Pension	Private Pension					

28

11 Other Insurances

It is sufficient to give an overview, since the documents are usually in a separate folder.

Type of Contract	Customer Number/ Contract Number	Contracting Party, Address, Telephone
Life Insurance #1		
Life Insurance #2		
Accident Insurance		
Repatriation-Insurance		
Occupational Disability Insurance		
Household Insurance		
Liability insurance		
Car Insurance		

12 Other Contracts

It is sufficient to give an overview, since the documents are usually in a separate folder.

Type of Contract	Customer Number/ Contract Number	Contracting Party, Address, Telephone
Landline Phone		
Mobile Phone		
Internet		
Subscription for …		

13 Real Estate (self-inhabited)

13.1 Real Estate (rented and self-inhabited)

Address and Location in the House	
Type of Property (Flat, House etc.)	
Landlord (Name, Address, Telephone)	
Property Management (Name, Address, Telephone)	
Rental Contract	☐ is attached ☐ is in the folder ....
Electricity Contract	☐ is attached ☐ is in the folder ....
	☐ is attached ☐ is in the folder ....

Note: In many countries the rental contract does not end with the death of the tenant, but passes to the heirs. These have to terminate the lease.

13.2 Real Estate (self-inhabited property)

Address and Location in the House	
Type of Property (Flat, House etc.)	
Legal owner according to land registry	
Name of financing Bank	
Property Management (Name, Address, Telephone)	
Electricity supplier	☐ Contract is attached ☐ Contract is in the folder ....
Other Suppliers (e.g. waste collection)	☐ Contract is attached ☐ Contract is in the folder ....

14 Real Estate (rented out)

It is sufficient to give an overview, since the documents are usually in separate folders.

Address and Location in the House	
Type of Property (Flat, House etc.)	
Legal owner according to land registry	
Name of financing Bank	
Name of Tenant(s)	
Telephone of Tenant(s)	
Property Management (Name, Address, Telephone)	

15 Mobile Assets

15.1 Cars, Boats, Aircraft etc.

What is it?	Registration	Location	Pitch Landlord	Insured at

15.2 Animals

Name + Type of Animal (e.g. Horse Balthazar)	Location	Insured at	Who should take care of it? (full Address + Telephone)	In Case of			
				Accident	Hospital stay	Death	

15.3 Permitted Weapons

In many countries weapons cannot be simply inherited. Often permitted weapons can only be inherited / given / sold to someone who has the required permissions or if they are permanently disabled. Otherwise, the heirs must hand in the weapons to the competent authority. Please inform yourself which authority is in charge in your country.

Attach here copies of the relevant documents/licenses and indicate the place where the weapons are stored:

____

____

____

____

16 Membership in Clubs, Societies, Associations etc.

Memberships in Clubs, Societies, Associations and other Institutions, which are to be terminated in the event of death.

Association etc.	Address	Membership Number

17 My digital legacy

A person's digital legacy is everything he leaves behind on his computer, his cell phone, his digital camera, his storage media or on the Internet or in companies. These data may be physically stored in different countries.

Overall, the young legal area "digital legacy" is still very confusing.

If you die your "accounts" will continue to exist on Facebook & Co, email providers and online shops etc. Your heirs do not have access to it. Even if the company disappears from the market due to bankruptcy, you must assume that the data will be taken over, evaluated or sold by any successor company.

If you (and your heirs) do not mind, you do not need to do anything. Maybe in 1,000 years, there is the profession of "digital archaeologist", who then researches these old databases to find out how the people of the 21st century lived.

However, if you want your data to be erased after death, you need to prepare accordingly.

- No matter what you want to do, an inventory of your digital activity is required first.
- One possibility is that your heirs use a death certificate or a certificate of inheritance to apply to your various providers for access to your accounts. However, this may take a long time because of the international nature of the topic, and perhaps not all providers will allow it.
- It is easier if you give your login data to a trusted friend and ask him to delete the stored data and close the accounts after your death. Nobody can delete your accounts if he does not know the login name and password.
- A more theoretical way is to delete accounts yourself, as long as you are still able to.

> **Of course it would be highly negligent to write down the login name _and_ password in one place. For if both go into unauthorized hands together, the contents of your accounts could be manipulated. In the case of bank accounts, you could even be robbed.**

Therefore: Always keep the login name and password separately !

Digital Activity	Login Name (User-ID)	What shall be done with it?
Example: www.doodle.com	max.miller@gmail.com	☐ delete it ☐ do nothing
		☐ delete it ☐ do nothing
		☐ delete it ☐ do nothing
		☐ delete it ☐ do nothing
		☐ delete it ☐ do nothing
		☐ delete it ☐ do nothing
		☐ delete it ☐ do nothing
		☐ delete it ☐ do nothing
		☐ delete it ☐ do nothing
		☐ delete it ☐ do nothing

18 My preventive power of attorney

Please insert here the original of your preventive power of attorney. If you insert a copy, please indicate where the original is located.

19 My care directive

Please insert here the original of your care directive. If you insert a copy, please indicate where the original is located.

52

20 My patient instruction

Please insert here the original of your patient instruction. If you insert a copy, please indicate where the original is located.

Please also include copies of any organ donation passports and tissue donation passports.

54

21 In the Event of Death

21.1 How to arrange my funeral

This section you have to formulate yourself (e.g. on the back side of this page). Often the will contains corresponding wishes / orders.

In any case, you should indicate here whether you have already commissioned a funeral home and whether you have already settled the costs of the funeral.

Name of Funeral Home	
Street, House number	
ZIP Code, City	
Telephone	
Place of contract details	
Costs prepaid?	☐ Yes ☐ No

21.2 Grave Speech

Bear in mind that the grave speaker often does not know the dead person well. To avoid that the grave speaker tells nonsense, you should feed him with information for a 10- to 15-minute speech. This includes at least the professional and personal CV, as well as a description of beloved persons and events that were important for your life.

The following notes can only be a suggestion:

- A professional CV usually describes schooling, education, and the different jobs.
- Which of the remaining friends come from the different phases of your life?
- In which phases did you meet or lose life partners?
- What do you want to say about your family(s)?
- What did you especially like to do or like?

- In which places did you enjoy living?
- Who would you like to thank?
- Who do you want to ask for forgiveness?

Only very few people will be able to write their eulogy in advance. So do not even try it. Individual paragraphs on the topics that are important to you will be sufficient.

Notes for the grave speech:

____

____

____

____

____

____

____

____

____

22 My Last Will

Here you can file the latest version of your will. If the will is not filed here, please indicate where it is kept (e.g. court, notary, friends)?

If you are worried that the first person to get your emergency folder in his hand will make the will disappear, you should file it with a court or notary.

For larger fortunes, assets abroad or probable inheritance disputes, it is recommended that the will be prepared and certified by a notary and possibly appoint an executor.

For optimum utilization of the tax-free allowances, inheritance planning by a tax advisor is recommended. Normally the heirs must transfer any inheritance tax that may be incurred to the tax authorities at very short notice. A forward-looking financial planning helps to avoid distress sales of assets e.g. real estate.

23 Me as a caregiver

You too could serve other people as a caregiver. Your relatives / friends / caregivers should be informed about this, because a substitute caregiver may have to step in.

I am caregiver for (Name, Address, Telephone)	Power of attorney
	☐ is attached ☐ is in the folder ....
	☐ is attached ☐ is in the folder ....
	☐ is attached ☐ is in the folder ....
	☐ is attached ☐ is in the folder ....
	☐ is attached ☐ is in the folder ....

24 Additional Notes

www.ingramcontent.com/pod-product-compliance
Lightning Source LLC
Chambersburg PA
CBHW081629250726
48657CB00009B/2797